THIS BOOK BELONGS TO:

CONTACT INFORMATION	
NAME:	
ADDRESS:	
PHONE:	

START / END DATES

___ / ___ / ___ TO ___ / ___ / ___

DEDICATION

This Juicing Journal Log book is dedicated to all the juicers out there who love to try new juices and smoothies and want to document their findings and favorite recipes in the process.

You are my inspiration for producing books and I'm honored to be a part of keeping all of your Juicing and Smoothie notes and recipes organized.

This journal notebook will help you record your recipes about trying new juices and smoothies.

Thoughtfully put together with these sections to record:

Prep Time, Juicing Time, Number of Ounces, Number of Servings, For Breakfast, Lunch, Dinner or Healing, Ingredients, How to Prepare, How I Felt, and Rating For This Juice.

HOW TO USE THIS BOOK

The purpose of this book is to keep all of your favorite Juicing and Smoothie recipes all in one place. It will help keep you organized.

This Juicing Journal will allow you to accurately document every detail about trying different juice and smoothie recipes. It's a great way to chart your course through juicing.

Here are examples of the prompts for you to fill in and write about your experience in this book:

1. **Prep Time** - How much time did it take you to prepare the juice.
2. **Juicing Time** - How much time did it take you to drink the juice or smoothie.
3. **Number of Ounces** - Record the number of ounces it made.
4. **Number of Servings** - Log the number of servings it will make.
5. **For Breakfast, Lunch, Dinner, or Healing** - Check boxes to write when you had it.
6. **Ingredients** - List the ingredients.
7. **How to Prepare** - For writing the process and method by which you made it.
8. **How I Felt** - What were the effects, how did it make you feel and any notes and details you want to remember.
9. **My Rating For This Juice Recipe** - Rate your recipe 1-10.

Enjoy!

JUICE RECIPE

PREP TIME		# OF OUNCES	
JUICING TIME		# OF SERVINGS	

JUICE IS FOR:

○ BREAKFAST   ○ LUNCH   ○ DINNER   ○ HEALING

INGREDIENTS

HOW TO PREPARE

HOW I FELT

MY RATING FOR THIS JUICE RECIPE   ○1 ○2 ○3 ○4 ○5 ○6 ○7 ○8 ○9 ○10

JUICE RECIPE

PREP TIME		# OF OUNCES	
JUICING TIME		# OF SERVINGS	

JUICE IS FOR:

○ BREAKFAST   ○ LUNCH   ○ DINNER   ○ HEALING

INGREDIENTS

HOW TO PREPARE

HOW I FELT

MY RATING FOR THIS JUICE RECIPE   ○1 ○2 ○3 ○4 ○5 ○6 ○7 ○8 ○9 ○10

JUICE RECIPE

PREP TIME		# OF OUNCES	
JUICING TIME		# OF SERVINGS	

JUICE IS FOR:

○ BREAKFAST   ○ LUNCH   ○ DINNER   ○ HEALING

INGREDIENTS

HOW TO PREPARE

HOW I FELT

MY RATING FOR THIS JUICE RECIPE   ○ 1 ○ 2 ○ 3 ○ 4 ○ 5 ○ 6 ○ 7 ○ 8 ○ 9 ○ 10

JUICE RECIPE

PREP TIME		# OF OUNCES	
JUICING TIME		# OF SERVINGS	

JUICE IS FOR:

○ BREAKFAST   ○ LUNCH   ○ DINNER   ○ HEALING

INGREDIENTS

_____

_____

_____

_____

_____

_____

_____

_____

HOW TO PREPARE

_____

_____

_____

_____

HOW I FELT

_____

_____

_____

_____

| MY RATING FOR THIS JUICE RECIPE | ○ 1 ○ 2 ○ 3 ○ 4 ○ 5 ○ 6 ○ 7 ○ 8 ○ 9 ○ 10 |

JUICE RECIPE

PREP TIME		# OF OUNCES	
JUICING TIME		# OF SERVINGS	

JUICE IS FOR:

○ BREAKFAST   ○ LUNCH   ○ DINNER   ○ HEALING

INGREDIENTS

_____
_____
_____
_____
_____
_____
_____
_____

HOW TO PREPARE

_____
_____
_____
_____

HOW I FELT

_____
_____
_____

MY RATING FOR THIS JUICE RECIPE   ○1 ○2 ○3 ○4 ○5 ○6 ○7 ○8 ○9 ○10

JUICE RECIPE

PREP TIME		# OF OUNCES	
JUICING TIME		# OF SERVINGS	

JUICE IS FOR:

○ BREAKFAST   ○ LUNCH   ○ DINNER   ○ HEALING

INGREDIENTS

_____

_____

_____

_____

_____

_____

_____

_____

HOW TO PREPARE

_____

_____

_____

_____

HOW I FELT

_____

_____

_____

| MY RATING FOR THIS JUICE RECIPE | ○1 ○2 ○3 ○4 ○5 ○6 ○7 ○8 ○9 ○10 |

JUICE RECIPE

PREP TIME		# OF OUNCES	
JUICING TIME		# OF SERVINGS	

JUICE IS FOR:

○ BREAKFAST   ○ LUNCH   ○ DINNER   ○ HEALING

INGREDIENTS

_____   _____
_____   _____
_____   _____
_____   _____
_____   _____
_____   _____
_____   _____
_____   _____

HOW TO PREPARE

_____
_____
_____
_____
_____

HOW I FELT

_____
_____
_____

| MY RATING FOR THIS JUICE RECIPE | ○1 ○2 ○3 ○4 ○5 ○6 ○7 ○8 ○9 ○10 |

JUICE RECIPE

PREP TIME		# OF OUNCES	
JUICING TIME		# OF SERVINGS	

JUICE IS FOR:

○ BREAKFAST   ○ LUNCH   ○ DINNER   ○ HEALING

INGREDIENTS

_____

_____

_____

_____

_____

_____

_____

HOW TO PREPARE

_____

_____

_____

_____

HOW I FELT

_____

_____

_____

| MY RATING FOR THIS JUICE RECIPE | ○1 ○2 ○3 ○4 ○5 ○6 ○7 ○8 ○9 ○10 |

JUICE RECIPE

PREP TIME		# OF OUNCES	
JUICING TIME		# OF SERVINGS	

JUICE IS FOR:

○ BREAKFAST   ○ LUNCH   ○ DINNER   ○ HEALING

INGREDIENTS

_____   _____
_____   _____
_____   _____
_____   _____
_____   _____
_____   _____
_____   _____

HOW TO PREPARE

_____
_____
_____
_____

HOW I FELT

_____
_____
_____

| MY RATING FOR THIS JUICE RECIPE | ○ 1 ○ 2 ○ 3 ○ 4 ○ 5 ○ 6 ○ 7 ○ 8 ○ 9 ○ 10 |

JUICE RECIPE

PREP TIME		# OF OUNCES	
JUICING TIME		# OF SERVINGS	

JUICE IS FOR:

○ BREAKFAST　　○ LUNCH　　○ DINNER　　○ HEALING

INGREDIENTS

_____
_____
_____
_____
_____
_____
_____
_____

HOW TO PREPARE

_____
_____
_____
_____

HOW I FELT

_____
_____
_____

MY RATING FOR THIS JUICE RECIPE　　○1　○2　○3　○4　○5　○6　○7　○8　○9　○10

JUICE RECIPE

PREP TIME		# OF OUNCES	
JUICING TIME		# OF SERVINGS	

JUICE IS FOR:

○ BREAKFAST   ○ LUNCH   ○ DINNER   ○ HEALING

INGREDIENTS

_____   _____
_____   _____
_____   _____
_____   _____
_____   _____
_____   _____
_____   _____
_____   _____

HOW TO PREPARE

_____
_____
_____
_____

HOW I FELT

_____
_____
_____

MY RATING FOR THIS JUICE RECIPE   ○ 1 ○ 2 ○ 3 ○ 4 ○ 5 ○ 6 ○ 7 ○ 8 ○ 9 ○ 10

JUICE RECIPE

PREP TIME		# OF OUNCES	
JUICING TIME		# OF SERVINGS	

JUICE IS FOR:

○ BREAKFAST   ○ LUNCH   ○ DINNER   ○ HEALING

INGREDIENTS

_____

_____

_____

_____

_____

_____

_____

_____

HOW TO PREPARE

_____

_____

_____

_____

HOW I FELT

_____

_____

_____

MY RATING FOR THIS JUICE RECIPE   ○1 ○2 ○3 ○4 ○5 ○6 ○7 ○8 ○9 ○10

JUICE RECIPE

PREP TIME		# OF OUNCES	
JUICING TIME		# OF SERVINGS	

JUICE IS FOR:			
○ BREAKFAST	○ LUNCH	○ DINNER	○ HEALING

INGREDIENTS

_____   _____
_____   _____
_____   _____
_____   _____
_____   _____
_____   _____
_____   _____
_____   _____

HOW TO PREPARE

_____
_____
_____
_____
_____

HOW I FELT

_____
_____
_____

MY RATING FOR THIS JUICE RECIPE	○ 1 ○ 2 ○ 3 ○ 4 ○ 5 ○ 6 ○ 7 ○ 8 ○ 9 ○ 10

JUICE RECIPE

PREP TIME		# OF OUNCES	
JUICING TIME		# OF SERVINGS	

JUICE IS FOR:

○ BREAKFAST   ○ LUNCH   ○ DINNER   ○ HEALING

INGREDIENTS

HOW TO PREPARE

HOW I FELT

MY RATING FOR THIS JUICE RECIPE   ○ 1 ○ 2 ○ 3 ○ 4 ○ 5 ○ 6 ○ 7 ○ 8 ○ 9 ○ 10

JUICE RECIPE

PREP TIME		# OF OUNCES	
JUICING TIME		# OF SERVINGS	

JUICE IS FOR:

○ BREAKFAST ○ LUNCH ○ DINNER ○ HEALING

INGREDIENTS

_____
_____
_____
_____
_____
_____
_____
_____

HOW TO PREPARE

_____
_____
_____
_____

HOW I FELT

_____
_____
_____

MY RATING FOR THIS JUICE RECIPE ○1 ○2 ○3 ○4 ○5 ○6 ○7 ○8 ○9 ○10

JUICE RECIPE

PREP TIME		# OF OUNCES	
JUICING TIME		# OF SERVINGS	

JUICE IS FOR:

○ BREAKFAST   ○ LUNCH   ○ DINNER   ○ HEALING

INGREDIENTS

_____

_____

_____

_____

_____

_____

_____

HOW TO PREPARE

_____

_____

_____

_____

HOW I FELT

_____

_____

_____

| MY RATING FOR THIS JUICE RECIPE | ○1 ○2 ○3 ○4 ○5 ○6 ○7 ○8 ○9 ○10 |

JUICE RECIPE

PREP TIME		# OF OUNCES	
JUICING TIME		# OF SERVINGS	

JUICE IS FOR:

○ BREAKFAST ○ LUNCH ○ DINNER ○ HEALING

INGREDIENTS

_____   _____
_____   _____
_____   _____
_____   _____
_____   _____
_____   _____
_____   _____
_____   _____

HOW TO PREPARE

_____
_____
_____
_____
_____

HOW I FELT

_____
_____
_____

MY RATING FOR THIS JUICE RECIPE   ○ 1 ○ 2 ○ 3 ○ 4 ○ 5 ○ 6 ○ 7 ○ 8 ○ 9 ○ 10

JUICE RECIPE

PREP TIME		# OF OUNCES	
JUICING TIME		# OF SERVINGS	

JUICE IS FOR:

○ BREAKFAST ○ LUNCH ○ DINNER ○ HEALING

INGREDIENTS

HOW TO PREPARE

HOW I FELT

MY RATING FOR THIS JUICE RECIPE ○1 ○2 ○3 ○4 ○5 ○6 ○7 ○8 ○9 ○10

JUICE RECIPE

PREP TIME		# OF OUNCES	
JUICING TIME		# OF SERVINGS	

JUICE IS FOR:

○ BREAKFAST　　　○ LUNCH　　　○ DINNER　　　○ HEALING

INGREDIENTS

_____　_____
_____　_____
_____　_____
_____　_____
_____　_____
_____　_____
_____　_____
_____　_____
_____　_____

HOW TO PREPARE

_____
_____
_____
_____
_____

HOW I FELT

_____
_____
_____

| MY RATING FOR THIS JUICE RECIPE | ○1　○2　○3　○4　○5　○6　○7　○8　○9　○10 |

JUICE RECIPE

PREP TIME		# OF OUNCES	
JUICING TIME		# OF SERVINGS	

JUICE IS FOR:

○ BREAKFAST ○ LUNCH ○ DINNER ○ HEALING

INGREDIENTS

HOW TO PREPARE

HOW I FELT

MY RATING FOR THIS JUICE RECIPE ○1 ○2 ○3 ○4 ○5 ○6 ○7 ○8 ○9 ○10

JUICE RECIPE

PREP TIME		# OF OUNCES	
JUICING TIME		# OF SERVINGS	

JUICE IS FOR:

○ BREAKFAST   ○ LUNCH   ○ DINNER   ○ HEALING

INGREDIENTS

_____

_____

_____

_____

_____

_____

_____

_____

HOW TO PREPARE

_____

_____

_____

_____

HOW I FELT

_____

_____

_____

MY RATING FOR THIS JUICE RECIPE   ○1 ○2 ○3 ○4 ○5 ○6 ○7 ○8 ○9 ○10

JUICE RECIPE

PREP TIME		# OF OUNCES	
JUICING TIME		# OF SERVINGS	

JUICE IS FOR:

○ BREAKFAST   ○ LUNCH   ○ DINNER   ○ HEALING

INGREDIENTS

HOW TO PREPARE

HOW I FELT

MY RATING FOR THIS JUICE RECIPE ○1 ○2 ○3 ○4 ○5 ○6 ○7 ○8 ○9 ○10

JUICE RECIPE

PREP TIME		# OF OUNCES	
JUICING TIME		# OF SERVINGS	

JUICE IS FOR:

○ BREAKFAST　　○ LUNCH　　○ DINNER　　○ HEALING

INGREDIENTS

_____   _____
_____   _____
_____   _____
_____   _____
_____   _____
_____   _____
_____   _____

HOW TO PREPARE

_____
_____
_____
_____
_____

HOW I FELT

_____
_____
_____

MY RATING FOR THIS JUICE RECIPE　　○1　○2　○3　○4　○5　○6　○7　○8　○9　○10

JUICE RECIPE

PREP TIME		# OF OUNCES	
JUICING TIME		# OF SERVINGS	

JUICE IS FOR:

○ BREAKFAST ○ LUNCH ○ DINNER ○ HEALING

INGREDIENTS

_____
_____
_____
_____
_____
_____
_____
_____

HOW TO PREPARE

_____
_____
_____
_____

HOW I FELT

_____
_____
_____

MY RATING FOR THIS JUICE RECIPE	○1 ○2 ○3 ○4 ○5 ○6 ○7 ○8 ○9 ○10

JUICE RECIPE

PREP TIME		# OF OUNCES	
JUICING TIME		# OF SERVINGS	

JUICE IS FOR:

○ BREAKFAST   ○ LUNCH   ○ DINNER   ○ HEALING

INGREDIENTS

_____   _____
_____   _____
_____   _____
_____   _____
_____   _____
_____   _____
_____   _____
_____   _____

HOW TO PREPARE

_____
_____
_____
_____

HOW I FELT

_____
_____
_____

| MY RATING FOR THIS JUICE RECIPE | ○1 ○2 ○3 ○4 ○5 ○6 ○7 ○8 ○9 ○10 |

JUICE RECIPE

PREP TIME		# OF OUNCES	
JUICING TIME		# OF SERVINGS	

JUICE IS FOR:

○ BREAKFAST   ○ LUNCH   ○ DINNER   ○ HEALING

INGREDIENTS

HOW TO PREPARE

HOW I FELT

MY RATING FOR THIS JUICE RECIPE   ○1 ○2 ○3 ○4 ○5 ○6 ○7 ○8 ○9 ○10

JUICE RECIPE

PREP TIME		# OF OUNCES	
JUICING TIME		# OF SERVINGS	

JUICE IS FOR:

○ BREAKFAST　　○ LUNCH　　○ DINNER　　○ HEALING

INGREDIENTS

_____
_____
_____
_____
_____
_____
_____
_____

HOW TO PREPARE

_____
_____
_____
_____

HOW I FELT

_____
_____
_____

MY RATING FOR THIS JUICE RECIPE　　○1　○2　○3　○4　○5　○6　○7　○8　○9　○10

JUICE RECIPE

PREP TIME		# OF OUNCES	
JUICING TIME		# OF SERVINGS	

JUICE IS FOR:

○ BREAKFAST ○ LUNCH ○ DINNER ○ HEALING

INGREDIENTS

HOW TO PREPARE

HOW I FELT

MY RATING FOR THIS JUICE RECIPE ○1 ○2 ○3 ○4 ○5 ○6 ○7 ○8 ○9 ○10

JUICE RECIPE

PREP TIME		# OF OUNCES	
JUICING TIME		# OF SERVINGS	

JUICE IS FOR:

○ BREAKFAST   ○ LUNCH   ○ DINNER   ○ HEALING

INGREDIENTS

_____   _____
_____   _____
_____   _____
_____   _____
_____   _____
_____   _____
_____   _____
_____   _____

HOW TO PREPARE

_____
_____
_____
_____
_____

HOW I FELT

_____
_____
_____

MY RATING FOR THIS JUICE RECIPE	○ 1 ○ 2 ○ 3 ○ 4 ○ 5 ○ 6 ○ 7 ○ 8 ○ 9 ○ 10

JUICE RECIPE

PREP TIME		# OF OUNCES	
JUICING TIME		# OF SERVINGS	

JUICE IS FOR:

○ BREAKFAST ○ LUNCH ○ DINNER ○ HEALING

INGREDIENTS

_____

_____

_____

_____

_____

_____

_____

HOW TO PREPARE

_____

_____

_____

_____

HOW I FELT

_____

_____

_____

| MY RATING FOR THIS JUICE RECIPE | ○1 ○2 ○3 ○4 ○5 ○6 ○7 ○8 ○9 ○10 |

JUICE RECIPE

PREP TIME		# OF OUNCES	
JUICING TIME		# OF SERVINGS	

JUICE IS FOR:

○ BREAKFAST ○ LUNCH ○ DINNER ○ HEALING

INGREDIENTS

HOW TO PREPARE

HOW I FELT

MY RATING FOR THIS JUICE RECIPE   ○1 ○2 ○3 ○4 ○5 ○6 ○7 ○8 ○9 ○10

JUICE RECIPE

PREP TIME		# OF OUNCES	
JUICING TIME		# OF SERVINGS	

JUICE IS FOR:

○ BREAKFAST　　○ LUNCH　　○ DINNER　　○ HEALING

INGREDIENTS

_____
_____
_____
_____
_____
_____
_____

HOW TO PREPARE

_____
_____
_____
_____

HOW I FELT

_____
_____
_____

MY RATING FOR THIS JUICE RECIPE	○ 1　○ 2　○ 3　○ 4　○ 5　○ 6　○ 7　○ 8　○ 9　○ 10

JUICE RECIPE

PREP TIME		# OF OUNCES	
JUICING TIME		# OF SERVINGS	

JUICE IS FOR:

○ BREAKFAST   ○ LUNCH   ○ DINNER   ○ HEALING

INGREDIENTS

HOW TO PREPARE

HOW I FELT

MY RATING FOR THIS JUICE RECIPE   ○ 1 ○ 2 ○ 3 ○ 4 ○ 5 ○ 6 ○ 7 ○ 8 ○ 9 ○ 10

JUICE RECIPE

PREP TIME		# OF OUNCES	
JUICING TIME		# OF SERVINGS	

JUICE IS FOR:

○ BREAKFAST ○ LUNCH ○ DINNER ○ HEALING

INGREDIENTS

HOW TO PREPARE

HOW I FELT

MY RATING FOR THIS JUICE RECIPE   ○ 1 ○ 2 ○ 3 ○ 4 ○ 5 ○ 6 ○ 7 ○ 8 ○ 9 ○ 10

JUICE RECIPE

PREP TIME		# OF OUNCES	
JUICING TIME		# OF SERVINGS	

JUICE IS FOR:

○ BREAKFAST   ○ LUNCH   ○ DINNER   ○ HEALING

INGREDIENTS

_____   _____
_____   _____
_____   _____
_____   _____
_____   _____
_____   _____
_____   _____

HOW TO PREPARE

_____
_____
_____
_____
_____

HOW I FELT

_____
_____
_____

MY RATING FOR THIS JUICE RECIPE   ○ 1 ○ 2 ○ 3 ○ 4 ○ 5 ○ 6 ○ 7 ○ 8 ○ 9 ○ 10

JUICE RECIPE

PREP TIME		# OF OUNCES	
JUICING TIME		# OF SERVINGS	

JUICE IS FOR:

○ BREAKFAST   ○ LUNCH   ○ DINNER   ○ HEALING

INGREDIENTS

_____

_____

_____

_____

_____

_____

_____

HOW TO PREPARE

_____

_____

_____

HOW I FELT

_____

_____

_____

MY RATING FOR THIS JUICE RECIPE	○1 ○2 ○3 ○4 ○5 ○6 ○7 ○8 ○9 ○10

JUICE RECIPE

PREP TIME		# OF OUNCES	
JUICING TIME		# OF SERVINGS	

JUICE IS FOR:

○ BREAKFAST   ○ LUNCH   ○ DINNER   ○ HEALING

INGREDIENTS

_____   _____
_____   _____
_____   _____
_____   _____
_____   _____
_____   _____
_____   _____
_____   _____

HOW TO PREPARE

_____
_____
_____
_____

HOW I FELT

_____
_____
_____

MY RATING FOR THIS JUICE RECIPE	○1 ○2 ○3 ○4 ○5 ○6 ○7 ○8 ○9 ○10

JUICE RECIPE

PREP TIME		# OF OUNCES	
JUICING TIME		# OF SERVINGS	

JUICE IS FOR:

○ BREAKFAST ○ LUNCH ○ DINNER ○ HEALING

INGREDIENTS

HOW TO PREPARE

HOW I FELT

MY RATING FOR THIS JUICE RECIPE ○1 ○2 ○3 ○4 ○5 ○6 ○7 ○8 ○9 ○10

JUICE RECIPE

PREP TIME		# OF OUNCES	
JUICING TIME		# OF SERVINGS	

JUICE IS FOR:

○ BREAKFAST   ○ LUNCH   ○ DINNER   ○ HEALING

INGREDIENTS

_____   _____
_____   _____
_____   _____
_____   _____
_____   _____
_____   _____
_____   _____

HOW TO PREPARE

_____
_____
_____
_____

HOW I FELT

_____
_____
_____

MY RATING FOR THIS JUICE RECIPE	○ 1 ○ 2 ○ 3 ○ 4 ○ 5 ○ 6 ○ 7 ○ 8 ○ 9 ○ 10

JUICE RECIPE

PREP TIME		# OF OUNCES	
JUICING TIME		# OF SERVINGS	

JUICE IS FOR:

○ BREAKFAST ○ LUNCH ○ DINNER ○ HEALING

INGREDIENTS

_____

_____

_____

_____

_____

_____

_____

_____

HOW TO PREPARE

_____

_____

_____

_____

HOW I FELT

_____

_____

_____

| MY RATING FOR THIS JUICE RECIPE | ○1 ○2 ○3 ○4 ○5 ○6 ○7 ○8 ○9 ○10 |

JUICE RECIPE

PREP TIME		# OF OUNCES	
JUICING TIME		# OF SERVINGS	

JUICE IS FOR:

○ BREAKFAST   ○ LUNCH   ○ DINNER   ○ HEALING

INGREDIENTS

_____

_____

_____

_____

_____

_____

_____

_____

_____

HOW TO PREPARE

_____

_____

_____

_____

_____

_____

HOW I FELT

_____

_____

_____

_____

| MY RATING FOR THIS JUICE RECIPE | ○ 1 ○ 2 ○ 3 ○ 4 ○ 5 ○ 6 ○ 7 ○ 8 ○ 9 ○ 10 |

JUICE RECIPE

PREP TIME		# OF OUNCES	
JUICING TIME		# OF SERVINGS	

JUICE IS FOR:

○ BREAKFAST   ○ LUNCH   ○ DINNER   ○ HEALING

INGREDIENTS

HOW TO PREPARE

HOW I FELT

| MY RATING FOR THIS JUICE RECIPE | ○ 1 ○ 2 ○ 3 ○ 4 ○ 5 ○ 6 ○ 7 ○ 8 ○ 9 ○ 10 |

JUICE RECIPE

PREP TIME		# OF OUNCES	
JUICING TIME		# OF SERVINGS	

JUICE IS FOR:			
○ BREAKFAST	○ LUNCH	○ DINNER	○ HEALING

INGREDIENTS

_____

_____

_____

_____

_____

_____

_____

_____

HOW TO PREPARE

_____

_____

_____

_____

HOW I FELT

_____

_____

_____

MY RATING FOR THIS JUICE RECIPE	○1 ○2 ○3 ○4 ○5 ○6 ○7 ○8 ○9 ○10

JUICE RECIPE

PREP TIME		# OF OUNCES	
JUICING TIME		# OF SERVINGS	

JUICE IS FOR:

○ BREAKFAST   ○ LUNCH   ○ DINNER   ○ HEALING

INGREDIENTS

HOW TO PREPARE

HOW I FELT

MY RATING FOR THIS JUICE RECIPE   ○1 ○2 ○3 ○4 ○5 ○6 ○7 ○8 ○9 ○10

JUICE RECIPE

PREP TIME		# OF OUNCES	
JUICING TIME		# OF SERVINGS	

JUICE IS FOR:

○ BREAKFAST   ○ LUNCH   ○ DINNER   ○ HEALING

INGREDIENTS

HOW TO PREPARE

HOW I FELT

MY RATING FOR THIS JUICE RECIPE   ○1 ○2 ○3 ○4 ○5 ○6 ○7 ○8 ○9 ○10

JUICE RECIPE

PREP TIME		# OF OUNCES	
JUICING TIME		# OF SERVINGS	

JUICE IS FOR:

○ BREAKFAST	○ LUNCH	○ DINNER	○ HEALING

INGREDIENTS

_____

_____

_____

_____

_____

_____

_____

_____

HOW TO PREPARE

_____

_____

_____

_____

HOW I FELT

_____

_____

_____

MY RATING FOR THIS JUICE RECIPE ○1 ○2 ○3 ○4 ○5 ○6 ○7 ○8 ○9 ○10

JUICE RECIPE

PREP TIME		# OF OUNCES	
JUICING TIME		# OF SERVINGS	

JUICE IS FOR:

○ BREAKFAST   ○ LUNCH   ○ DINNER   ○ HEALING

INGREDIENTS

_____

_____

_____

_____

_____

_____

_____

_____

HOW TO PREPARE

_____

_____

_____

_____

HOW I FELT

_____

_____

_____

MY RATING FOR THIS JUICE RECIPE   ○ 1   ○ 2   ○ 3   ○ 4   ○ 5   ○ 6   ○ 7   ○ 8   ○ 9   ○ 10

JUICE RECIPE

PREP TIME		# OF OUNCES	
JUICING TIME		# OF SERVINGS	

JUICE IS FOR:

○ BREAKFAST ○ LUNCH ○ DINNER ○ HEALING

INGREDIENTS

HOW TO PREPARE

HOW I FELT

MY RATING FOR THIS JUICE RECIPE   ○ 1 ○ 2 ○ 3 ○ 4 ○ 5 ○ 6 ○ 7 ○ 8 ○ 9 ○ 10

JUICE RECIPE

PREP TIME		# OF OUNCES	
JUICING TIME		# OF SERVINGS	

JUICE IS FOR:

○ BREAKFAST   ○ LUNCH   ○ DINNER   ○ HEALING

INGREDIENTS

HOW TO PREPARE

HOW I FELT

MY RATING FOR THIS JUICE RECIPE   ○1 ○2 ○3 ○4 ○5 ○6 ○7 ○8 ○9 ○10

JUICE RECIPE

PREP TIME		# OF OUNCES	
JUICING TIME		# OF SERVINGS	

JUICE IS FOR:

○ BREAKFAST   ○ LUNCH   ○ DINNER   ○ HEALING

INGREDIENTS

HOW TO PREPARE

HOW I FELT

MY RATING FOR THIS JUICE RECIPE   ○ 1 ○ 2 ○ 3 ○ 4 ○ 5 ○ 6 ○ 7 ○ 8 ○ 9 ○ 10

JUICE RECIPE

PREP TIME		# OF OUNCES	
JUICING TIME		# OF SERVINGS	

JUICE IS FOR:

○ BREAKFAST   ○ LUNCH   ○ DINNER   ○ HEALING

INGREDIENTS

_____   _____
_____   _____
_____   _____
_____   _____
_____   _____
_____   _____
_____   _____

HOW TO PREPARE

_____
_____
_____
_____
_____

HOW I FELT

_____
_____
_____

MY RATING FOR THIS JUICE RECIPE   ○1 ○2 ○3 ○4 ○5 ○6 ○7 ○8 ○9 ○10

JUICE RECIPE

PREP TIME		# OF OUNCES	
JUICING TIME		# OF SERVINGS	

JUICE IS FOR:

○ BREAKFAST   ○ LUNCH   ○ DINNER   ○ HEALING

INGREDIENTS

_____
_____
_____
_____
_____
_____
_____

HOW TO PREPARE

_____
_____
_____
_____

HOW I FELT

_____
_____
_____

MY RATING FOR THIS JUICE RECIPE	○1 ○2 ○3 ○4 ○5 ○6 ○7 ○8 ○9 ○10

JUICE RECIPE

PREP TIME		# OF OUNCES	
JUICING TIME		# OF SERVINGS	

JUICE IS FOR:

○ BREAKFAST ○ LUNCH ○ DINNER ○ HEALING

INGREDIENTS

_____
_____
_____
_____
_____
_____
_____
_____

HOW TO PREPARE

_____
_____
_____
_____
_____

HOW I FELT

_____
_____
_____

MY RATING FOR THIS JUICE RECIPE   ○1 ○2 ○3 ○4 ○5 ○6 ○7 ○8 ○9 ○10

JUICE RECIPE

PREP TIME		# OF OUNCES	
JUICING TIME		# OF SERVINGS	

JUICE IS FOR:

○ BREAKFAST   ○ LUNCH   ○ DINNER   ○ HEALING

INGREDIENTS

HOW TO PREPARE

HOW I FELT

MY RATING FOR THIS JUICE RECIPE   ○1 ○2 ○3 ○4 ○5 ○6 ○7 ○8 ○9 ○10

JUICE RECIPE

PREP TIME		# OF OUNCES	
JUICING TIME		# OF SERVINGS	

JUICE IS FOR:

○ BREAKFAST   ○ LUNCH   ○ DINNER   ○ HEALING

INGREDIENTS

_____

_____

_____

_____

_____

_____

_____

_____

_____

HOW TO PREPARE

_____

_____

_____

_____

HOW I FELT

_____

_____

_____

| MY RATING FOR THIS JUICE RECIPE | ○1 ○2 ○3 ○4 ○5 ○6 ○7 ○8 ○9 ○10 |

JUICE RECIPE

PREP TIME		# OF OUNCES	
JUICING TIME		# OF SERVINGS	

JUICE IS FOR:

○ BREAKFAST　　○ LUNCH　　○ DINNER　　○ HEALING

INGREDIENTS

HOW TO PREPARE

HOW I FELT

| MY RATING FOR THIS JUICE RECIPE | ○1　○2　○3　○4　○5　○6　○7　○8　○9　○10 |

JUICE RECIPE

PREP TIME		# OF OUNCES	
JUICING TIME		# OF SERVINGS	

JUICE IS FOR:

○ BREAKFAST   ○ LUNCH   ○ DINNER   ○ HEALING

INGREDIENTS

HOW TO PREPARE

HOW I FELT

MY RATING FOR THIS JUICE RECIPE   ○ 1 ○ 2 ○ 3 ○ 4 ○ 5 ○ 6 ○ 7 ○ 8 ○ 9 ○ 10

JUICE RECIPE

PREP TIME		# OF OUNCES	
JUICING TIME		# OF SERVINGS	

JUICE IS FOR:

○ BREAKFAST   ○ LUNCH   ○ DINNER   ○ HEALING

INGREDIENTS

_____   _____
_____   _____
_____   _____
_____   _____
_____   _____
_____   _____
_____   _____

HOW TO PREPARE

_____
_____
_____
_____

HOW I FELT

_____
_____
_____

MY RATING FOR THIS JUICE RECIPE	○1 ○2 ○3 ○4 ○5 ○6 ○7 ○8 ○9 ○10

JUICE RECIPE

PREP TIME		# OF OUNCES	
JUICING TIME		# OF SERVINGS	

JUICE IS FOR:

○ BREAKFAST　　　○ LUNCH　　　○ DINNER　　　○ HEALING

INGREDIENTS

_____

_____

_____

_____

_____

_____

_____

_____

HOW TO PREPARE

_____

_____

_____

_____

HOW I FELT

_____

_____

_____

| MY RATING FOR THIS JUICE RECIPE | ○ 1　○ 2　○ 3　○ 4　○ 5　○ 6　○ 7　○ 8　○ 9　○ 10 |

JUICE RECIPE

PREP TIME		# OF OUNCES	
JUICING TIME		# OF SERVINGS	

JUICE IS FOR:

○ BREAKFAST   ○ LUNCH   ○ DINNER   ○ HEALING

INGREDIENTS

_____
_____
_____
_____
_____
_____
_____
_____

HOW TO PREPARE

_____
_____
_____
_____

HOW I FELT

_____
_____
_____

| MY RATING FOR THIS JUICE RECIPE | ○1 ○2 ○3 ○4 ○5 ○6 ○7 ○8 ○9 ○10 |

JUICE RECIPE

PREP TIME		# OF OUNCES	
JUICING TIME		# OF SERVINGS	

JUICE IS FOR:

○ BREAKFAST ○ LUNCH ○ DINNER ○ HEALING

INGREDIENTS

HOW TO PREPARE

HOW I FELT

MY RATING FOR THIS JUICE RECIPE   ○1 ○2 ○3 ○4 ○5 ○6 ○7 ○8 ○9 ○10

JUICE RECIPE

PREP TIME		# OF OUNCES	
JUICING TIME		# OF SERVINGS	

JUICE IS FOR:

○ BREAKFAST　　○ LUNCH　　○ DINNER　　○ HEALING

INGREDIENTS

HOW TO PREPARE

HOW I FELT

MY RATING FOR THIS JUICE RECIPE　　○1　○2　○3　○4　○5　○6　○7　○8　○9　○10

JUICE RECIPE

PREP TIME		# OF OUNCES	
JUICING TIME		# OF SERVINGS	

JUICE IS FOR:

○ BREAKFAST　　○ LUNCH　　○ DINNER　　○ HEALING

INGREDIENTS

_____

_____

_____

_____

_____

_____

_____

_____

HOW TO PREPARE

_____

_____

_____

_____

HOW I FELT

_____

_____

_____

MY RATING FOR THIS JUICE RECIPE　　○1 ○2 ○3 ○4 ○5 ○6 ○7 ○8 ○9 ○10

JUICE RECIPE

PREP TIME		# OF OUNCES	
JUICING TIME		# OF SERVINGS	

JUICE IS FOR:

○ BREAKFAST   ○ LUNCH   ○ DINNER   ○ HEALING

INGREDIENTS

HOW TO PREPARE

HOW I FELT

MY RATING FOR THIS JUICE RECIPE   ○1 ○2 ○3 ○4 ○5 ○6 ○7 ○8 ○9 ○10

JUICE RECIPE

PREP TIME		# OF OUNCES	
JUICING TIME		# OF SERVINGS	

JUICE IS FOR:

○ BREAKFAST   ○ LUNCH   ○ DINNER   ○ HEALING

INGREDIENTS

_____   _____
_____   _____
_____   _____
_____   _____
_____   _____
_____   _____
_____   _____
_____   _____

HOW TO PREPARE

_____
_____
_____
_____
_____

HOW I FELT

_____
_____
_____

MY RATING FOR THIS JUICE RECIPE   ○1 ○2 ○3 ○4 ○5 ○6 ○7 ○8 ○9 ○10

JUICE RECIPE

PREP TIME		# OF OUNCES	
JUICING TIME		# OF SERVINGS	

JUICE IS FOR:

○ BREAKFAST　　○ LUNCH　　○ DINNER　　○ HEALING

INGREDIENTS

HOW TO PREPARE

HOW I FELT

MY RATING FOR THIS JUICE RECIPE　　○1　○2　○3　○4　○5　○6　○7　○8　○9　○10

JUICE RECIPE

PREP TIME		# OF OUNCES	
JUICING TIME		# OF SERVINGS	

JUICE IS FOR:

○ BREAKFAST   ○ LUNCH   ○ DINNER   ○ HEALING

INGREDIENTS

HOW TO PREPARE

HOW I FELT

MY RATING FOR THIS JUICE RECIPE   ○ 1 ○ 2 ○ 3 ○ 4 ○ 5 ○ 6 ○ 7 ○ 8 ○ 9 ○ 10

JUICE RECIPE

PREP TIME		# OF OUNCES	
JUICING TIME		# OF SERVINGS	

JUICE IS FOR:

○ BREAKFAST　　○ LUNCH　　○ DINNER　　○ HEALING

INGREDIENTS

_____
_____
_____
_____
_____
_____
_____

HOW TO PREPARE

_____
_____
_____
_____

HOW I FELT

_____
_____
_____

| MY RATING FOR THIS JUICE RECIPE | ○1　○2　○3　○4　○5　○6　○7　○8　○9　○10 |

JUICE RECIPE

PREP TIME		# OF OUNCES	
JUICING TIME		# OF SERVINGS	

JUICE IS FOR:

○ BREAKFAST   ○ LUNCH   ○ DINNER   ○ HEALING

INGREDIENTS

_____   _____
_____   _____
_____   _____
_____   _____
_____   _____
_____   _____
_____   _____

HOW TO PREPARE

_____
_____
_____
_____

HOW I FELT

_____
_____
_____

MY RATING FOR THIS JUICE RECIPE	○ 1 ○ 2 ○ 3 ○ 4 ○ 5 ○ 6 ○ 7 ○ 8 ○ 9 ○ 10

JUICE RECIPE

PREP TIME		# OF OUNCES	
JUICING TIME		# OF SERVINGS	

JUICE IS FOR:

○ BREAKFAST	○ LUNCH	○ DINNER	○ HEALING

INGREDIENTS

_____

_____

_____

_____

_____

_____

_____

HOW TO PREPARE

_____

_____

_____

_____

HOW I FELT

_____

_____

_____

MY RATING FOR THIS JUICE RECIPE	○ 1 ○ 2 ○ 3 ○ 4 ○ 5 ○ 6 ○ 7 ○ 8 ○ 9 ○ 10

JUICE RECIPE

PREP TIME		# OF OUNCES	
JUICING TIME		# OF SERVINGS	

JUICE IS FOR:

○ BREAKFAST   ○ LUNCH   ○ DINNER   ○ HEALING

INGREDIENTS

_____   _____
_____   _____
_____   _____
_____   _____
_____   _____
_____   _____
_____   _____
_____   _____

HOW TO PREPARE

_____
_____
_____
_____
_____

HOW I FELT

_____
_____
_____

MY RATING FOR THIS JUICE RECIPE   ○ 1 ○ 2 ○ 3 ○ 4 ○ 5 ○ 6 ○ 7 ○ 8 ○ 9 ○ 10

JUICE RECIPE

PREP TIME		# OF OUNCES	
JUICING TIME		# OF SERVINGS	

JUICE IS FOR:

○ BREAKFAST	○ LUNCH	○ DINNER	○ HEALING

INGREDIENTS

HOW TO PREPARE

HOW I FELT

MY RATING FOR THIS JUICE RECIPE   ○1 ○2 ○3 ○4 ○5 ○6 ○7 ○8 ○9 ○10

JUICE RECIPE

PREP TIME		# OF OUNCES	
JUICING TIME		# OF SERVINGS	

JUICE IS FOR:

○ BREAKFAST   ○ LUNCH   ○ DINNER   ○ HEALING

INGREDIENTS

HOW TO PREPARE

HOW I FELT

MY RATING FOR THIS JUICE RECIPE   ○ 1 ○ 2 ○ 3 ○ 4 ○ 5 ○ 6 ○ 7 ○ 8 ○ 9 ○ 10

JUICE RECIPE

PREP TIME		# OF OUNCES	
JUICING TIME		# OF SERVINGS	

JUICE IS FOR:

○ BREAKFAST   ○ LUNCH   ○ DINNER   ○ HEALING

INGREDIENTS

HOW TO PREPARE

HOW I FELT

MY RATING FOR THIS JUICE RECIPE   ○1 ○2 ○3 ○4 ○5 ○6 ○7 ○8 ○9 ○10

JUICE RECIPE

PREP TIME		# OF OUNCES	
JUICING TIME		# OF SERVINGS	

JUICE IS FOR:

○ BREAKFAST   ○ LUNCH   ○ DINNER   ○ HEALING

INGREDIENTS

___

HOW TO PREPARE

___

HOW I FELT

___

MY RATING FOR THIS JUICE RECIPE   ○1 ○2 ○3 ○4 ○5 ○6 ○7 ○8 ○9 ○10

JUICE RECIPE

PREP TIME		# OF OUNCES	
JUICING TIME		# OF SERVINGS	

JUICE IS FOR:

○ BREAKFAST   ○ LUNCH   ○ DINNER   ○ HEALING

INGREDIENTS

_____

_____

_____

_____

_____

_____

_____

HOW TO PREPARE

_____

_____

_____

_____

HOW I FELT

_____

_____

_____

MY RATING FOR THIS JUICE RECIPE   ○1 ○2 ○3 ○4 ○5 ○6 ○7 ○8 ○9 ○10

JUICE RECIPE

PREP TIME		# OF OUNCES	
JUICING TIME		# OF SERVINGS	

JUICE IS FOR:

○ BREAKFAST   ○ LUNCH   ○ DINNER   ○ HEALING

INGREDIENTS

_____   _____
_____   _____
_____   _____
_____   _____
_____   _____
_____   _____
_____   _____
_____   _____

HOW TO PREPARE

_____
_____
_____
_____
_____

HOW I FELT

_____
_____
_____

| MY RATING FOR THIS JUICE RECIPE | ○ 1 ○ 2 ○ 3 ○ 4 ○ 5 ○ 6 ○ 7 ○ 8 ○ 9 ○ 10 |

JUICE RECIPE

PREP TIME		# OF OUNCES	
JUICING TIME		# OF SERVINGS	

JUICE IS FOR:

○ BREAKFAST ○ LUNCH ○ DINNER ○ HEALING

INGREDIENTS

_____

_____

_____

_____

_____

_____

_____

_____

HOW TO PREPARE

_____

_____

_____

_____

HOW I FELT

_____

_____

_____

MY RATING FOR THIS JUICE RECIPE   ○ 1 ○ 2 ○ 3 ○ 4 ○ 5 ○ 6 ○ 7 ○ 8 ○ 9 ○ 10

JUICE RECIPE

PREP TIME		# OF OUNCES	
JUICING TIME		# OF SERVINGS	

JUICE IS FOR:

○ BREAKFAST   ○ LUNCH   ○ DINNER   ○ HEALING

INGREDIENTS

_____   _____
_____   _____
_____   _____
_____   _____
_____   _____
_____   _____
_____   _____
_____   _____

HOW TO PREPARE

_____
_____
_____
_____
_____

HOW I FELT

_____
_____
_____

MY RATING FOR THIS JUICE RECIPE   ○ 1 ○ 2 ○ 3 ○ 4 ○ 5 ○ 6 ○ 7 ○ 8 ○ 9 ○ 10

JUICE RECIPE

PREP TIME		# OF OUNCES	
JUICING TIME		# OF SERVINGS	

JUICE IS FOR:

○ BREAKFAST   ○ LUNCH   ○ DINNER   ○ HEALING

INGREDIENTS

HOW TO PREPARE

HOW I FELT

MY RATING FOR THIS JUICE RECIPE ○1 ○2 ○3 ○4 ○5 ○6 ○7 ○8 ○9 ○10

JUICE RECIPE

PREP TIME		# OF OUNCES	
JUICING TIME		# OF SERVINGS	

JUICE IS FOR:

○ BREAKFAST　　○ LUNCH　　○ DINNER　　○ HEALING

INGREDIENTS

_____
_____
_____
_____
_____
_____
_____
_____

HOW TO PREPARE

_____
_____
_____
_____

HOW I FELT

_____
_____

MY RATING FOR THIS JUICE RECIPE　　○ 1　○ 2　○ 3　○ 4　○ 5　○ 6　○ 7　○ 8　○ 9　○ 10

JUICE RECIPE

PREP TIME		# OF OUNCES	
JUICING TIME		# OF SERVINGS	

JUICE IS FOR:

○ BREAKFAST ○ LUNCH ○ DINNER ○ HEALING

INGREDIENTS

HOW TO PREPARE

HOW I FELT

MY RATING FOR THIS JUICE RECIPE ○1 ○2 ○3 ○4 ○5 ○6 ○7 ○8 ○9 ○10

JUICE RECIPE

PREP TIME		# OF OUNCES	
JUICING TIME		# OF SERVINGS	

JUICE IS FOR:

○ BREAKFAST   ○ LUNCH   ○ DINNER   ○ HEALING

INGREDIENTS

HOW TO PREPARE

HOW I FELT

MY RATING FOR THIS JUICE RECIPE   ○1 ○2 ○3 ○4 ○5 ○6 ○7 ○8 ○9 ○10

JUICE RECIPE

PREP TIME		# OF OUNCES	
JUICING TIME		# OF SERVINGS	

JUICE IS FOR:

○ BREAKFAST   ○ LUNCH   ○ DINNER   ○ HEALING

INGREDIENTS

_____

_____

_____

_____

_____

_____

_____

HOW TO PREPARE

_____

_____

_____

_____

HOW I FELT

_____

_____

_____

| MY RATING FOR THIS JUICE RECIPE | ○1 ○2 ○3 ○4 ○5 ○6 ○7 ○8 ○9 ○10 |

JUICE RECIPE

PREP TIME		# OF OUNCES	
JUICING TIME		# OF SERVINGS	

JUICE IS FOR:

○ BREAKFAST ○ LUNCH ○ DINNER ○ HEALING

INGREDIENTS

HOW TO PREPARE

HOW I FELT

MY RATING FOR THIS JUICE RECIPE ○ 1 ○ 2 ○ 3 ○ 4 ○ 5 ○ 6 ○ 7 ○ 8 ○ 9 ○ 10

JUICE RECIPE

PREP TIME		# OF OUNCES	
JUICING TIME		# OF SERVINGS	

JUICE IS FOR:

○ BREAKFAST   ○ LUNCH   ○ DINNER   ○ HEALING

INGREDIENTS

HOW TO PREPARE

HOW I FELT

MY RATING FOR THIS JUICE RECIPE   ○ 1 ○ 2 ○ 3 ○ 4 ○ 5 ○ 6 ○ 7 ○ 8 ○ 9 ○ 10

JUICE RECIPE

PREP TIME		# OF OUNCES	
JUICING TIME		# OF SERVINGS	

JUICE IS FOR:

○ BREAKFAST   ○ LUNCH   ○ DINNER   ○ HEALING

INGREDIENTS

_____   _____
_____   _____
_____   _____
_____   _____
_____   _____
_____   _____
_____   _____
_____   _____

HOW TO PREPARE

_____
_____
_____
_____
_____

HOW I FELT

_____
_____
_____

MY RATING FOR THIS JUICE RECIPE   ○1 ○2 ○3 ○4 ○5 ○6 ○7 ○8 ○9 ○10

JUICE RECIPE

PREP TIME		# OF OUNCES	
JUICING TIME		# OF SERVINGS	

JUICE IS FOR:

○ BREAKFAST   ○ LUNCH   ○ DINNER   ○ HEALING

INGREDIENTS

HOW TO PREPARE

HOW I FELT

MY RATING FOR THIS JUICE RECIPE   ○ 1 ○ 2 ○ 3 ○ 4 ○ 5 ○ 6 ○ 7 ○ 8 ○ 9 ○ 10

JUICE RECIPE

PREP TIME		# OF OUNCES	
JUICING TIME		# OF SERVINGS	

JUICE IS FOR:

○ BREAKFAST   ○ LUNCH   ○ DINNER   ○ HEALING

INGREDIENTS

_____   _____
_____   _____
_____   _____
_____   _____
_____   _____
_____   _____
_____   _____
_____   _____

HOW TO PREPARE

_____
_____
_____
_____
_____

HOW I FELT

_____
_____
_____

| MY RATING FOR THIS JUICE RECIPE | ○1 ○2 ○3 ○4 ○5 ○6 ○7 ○8 ○9 ○10 |

JUICE RECIPE

PREP TIME		# OF OUNCES	
JUICING TIME		# OF SERVINGS	

JUICE IS FOR:

○ BREAKFAST ○ LUNCH ○ DINNER ○ HEALING

INGREDIENTS

___

HOW TO PREPARE

___

HOW I FELT

___

MY RATING FOR THIS JUICE RECIPE ○1 ○2 ○3 ○4 ○5 ○6 ○7 ○8 ○9 ○10

JUICE RECIPE

PREP TIME		# OF OUNCES	
JUICING TIME		# OF SERVINGS	

JUICE IS FOR:

○ BREAKFAST　　　○ LUNCH　　　○ DINNER　　　○ HEALING

INGREDIENTS

_____   _____
_____   _____
_____   _____
_____   _____
_____   _____
_____   _____
_____   _____
_____   _____

HOW TO PREPARE

_____
_____
_____
_____
_____

HOW I FELT

_____
_____
_____

MY RATING FOR THIS JUICE RECIPE　　○ 1　○ 2　○ 3　○ 4　○ 5　○ 6　○ 7　○ 8　○ 9　○ 10

JUICE RECIPE

PREP TIME		# OF OUNCES	
JUICING TIME		# OF SERVINGS	

JUICE IS FOR:

○ BREAKFAST   ○ LUNCH   ○ DINNER   ○ HEALING

INGREDIENTS

HOW TO PREPARE

HOW I FELT

MY RATING FOR THIS JUICE RECIPE   ○ 1 ○ 2 ○ 3 ○ 4 ○ 5 ○ 6 ○ 7 ○ 8 ○ 9 ○ 10

JUICE RECIPE

PREP TIME		# OF OUNCES	
JUICING TIME		# OF SERVINGS	

JUICE IS FOR:

○ BREAKFAST　　○ LUNCH　　○ DINNER　　○ HEALING

INGREDIENTS

_____　　_____
_____　　_____
_____　　_____
_____　　_____
_____　　_____
_____　　_____
_____　　_____

HOW TO PREPARE

_____
_____
_____
_____
_____

HOW I FELT

_____
_____
_____

MY RATING FOR THIS JUICE RECIPE　　○1　○2　○3　○4　○5　○6　○7　○8　○9　○10

JUICE RECIPE

PREP TIME		# OF OUNCES	
JUICING TIME		# OF SERVINGS	

JUICE IS FOR:

○ BREAKFAST   ○ LUNCH   ○ DINNER   ○ HEALING

INGREDIENTS

HOW TO PREPARE

HOW I FELT

MY RATING FOR THIS JUICE RECIPE   ○1 ○2 ○3 ○4 ○5 ○6 ○7 ○8 ○9 ○10

JUICE RECIPE

PREP TIME		# OF OUNCES	
JUICING TIME		# OF SERVINGS	

JUICE IS FOR:

○ BREAKFAST   ○ LUNCH   ○ DINNER   ○ HEALING

INGREDIENTS

_____   _____
_____   _____
_____   _____
_____   _____
_____   _____
_____   _____
_____   _____
_____   _____

HOW TO PREPARE

_____
_____
_____
_____
_____

HOW I FELT

_____
_____
_____

MY RATING FOR THIS JUICE RECIPE	○ 1 ○ 2 ○ 3 ○ 4 ○ 5 ○ 6 ○ 7 ○ 8 ○ 9 ○ 10

JUICE RECIPE

PREP TIME		# OF OUNCES	
JUICING TIME		# OF SERVINGS	

JUICE IS FOR:

○ BREAKFAST   ○ LUNCH   ○ DINNER   ○ HEALING

INGREDIENTS

_____

_____

_____

_____

_____

_____

_____

_____

HOW TO PREPARE

_____

_____

_____

_____

HOW I FELT

_____

_____

_____

MY RATING FOR THIS JUICE RECIPE   ○1 ○2 ○3 ○4 ○5 ○6 ○7 ○8 ○9 ○10

JUICE RECIPE

PREP TIME		# OF OUNCES	
JUICING TIME		# OF SERVINGS	

JUICE IS FOR:

○ BREAKFAST   ○ LUNCH   ○ DINNER   ○ HEALING

INGREDIENTS

HOW TO PREPARE

HOW I FELT

MY RATING FOR THIS JUICE RECIPE   ○ 1 ○ 2 ○ 3 ○ 4 ○ 5 ○ 6 ○ 7 ○ 8 ○ 9 ○ 10

JUICE RECIPE

PREP TIME		# OF OUNCES	
JUICING TIME		# OF SERVINGS	

JUICE IS FOR:

○ BREAKFAST ○ LUNCH ○ DINNER ○ HEALING

INGREDIENTS

HOW TO PREPARE

HOW I FELT

MY RATING FOR THIS JUICE RECIPE   ○1 ○2 ○3 ○4 ○5 ○6 ○7 ○8 ○9 ○10

JUICE RECIPE

PREP TIME		# OF OUNCES	
JUICING TIME		# OF SERVINGS	

JUICE IS FOR:

○ BREAKFAST　　○ LUNCH　　○ DINNER　　○ HEALING

INGREDIENTS

_____　　_____
_____　　_____
_____　　_____
_____　　_____
_____　　_____
_____　　_____
_____　　_____

HOW TO PREPARE

_____
_____
_____
_____

HOW I FELT

_____
_____
_____

MY RATING FOR THIS JUICE RECIPE　　○1　○2　○3　○4　○5　○6　○7　○8　○9　○10

JUICE RECIPE

PREP TIME		# OF OUNCES	
JUICING TIME		# OF SERVINGS	

JUICE IS FOR:

○ BREAKFAST   ○ LUNCH   ○ DINNER   ○ HEALING

INGREDIENTS

_____

_____

_____

_____

_____

_____

_____

HOW TO PREPARE

_____

_____

_____

HOW I FELT

_____

_____

_____

MY RATING FOR THIS JUICE RECIPE	○1 ○2 ○3 ○4 ○5 ○6 ○7 ○8 ○9 ○10

JUICE RECIPE

PREP TIME		# OF OUNCES	
JUICING TIME		# OF SERVINGS	

JUICE IS FOR:

○ BREAKFAST   ○ LUNCH   ○ DINNER   ○ HEALING

INGREDIENTS

HOW TO PREPARE

HOW I FELT

MY RATING FOR THIS JUICE RECIPE   ○ 1   ○ 2   ○ 3   ○ 4   ○ 5   ○ 6   ○ 7   ○ 8   ○ 9   ○ 10